The Ehler Danlos Patient's Sourcebook

Paul Kalman, MA

Johnson White, MD (Ed.)

ISBN: 978-1503224407

Contents

INTRODUCTION

Ehlers-Danlos Syndrome (EDS) affects the connective tissues; the joint and skin problems are due to issues with collagen, proteins that stabilize the connective tissue and give it elasticity. Prior to 1997, there were 10 recognized types of EDS which were classified by Roman numerals (e.g. EDS I , II and III), but this has now been simplified to six major types:

- The arthrochalasia type
- The classic type
- The dermatosparaxis type
- The hypermobility type
- The kyphoscoliosis type
- The vascular type.

Each type has its own features. For example, the vascular type of Ehlers-Danlos syndrome carries an increased risk of organ rupture, including tearing of the aorta and rupture of the uterus (womb) during pregnancy. All types have some effect on the joints, with symptoms that typically include:

- Ability to over extend joints (hyperextension)
- Chronic pain in joints
- Early onset osteoarthritis
- Fragile skin, blood vessels, membranes and other tissues
- Loose and elastic skin
- Loose joints (laxity)
- Poor wound healing
- Prolonged bleeding following cuts or other trauma
- Scars that are thinner than usual (parchment-like)
- Tendency to bruise easily
- Tendency to dislocate joints

EDS is a hereditary disorder that runs in families. Each of the six subtypes is a distinct entity, so families will tend to only have one subtype. For example, parents with the classic type of EDS will not have children with the hypermobility type.

Symptoms may first show up during the childhood years, although some newborns with certain subtypes are diagnosed with EDS. If symptoms are mild, the disorder may not be diagnosed until the adult years.

Males and females are equally affected by EDS, with the exception of an X-linked EDS subtype which only affects males. It is thought that between one in 5,000 and one in 10,000 children are born with the condition. However, exact numbers are not known.

Types

Classical Type

The classical type of EDS can be mild or it can be severe. The original Roman numeral system differentiated between mild (EDS I) and severe (EDS II) variations, but the new, simpler classification system recognized both variations as the same, classical type. People with EDS classical type have a wide variation in skin abnormalities which may range from mild to severe (Kindreds).

Symptoms usually include:
- Abnormal healing wounds
- Dislocated joints (especially knees and shoulders)
- Fragile skin that can sometimes split easily
- Frequent sprains
- Overly elastic skin (hyperextensibility of the skin)

- Thin, paper-like scarring, especially over elbows, forehead, shins and knees
- Unusual ability to over-extend joints (hypermobility).

Some people with classical EDS have less common signs and symptoms, including:
- Molluscoid pseudotumors: small, flesh-like skin growths
- calcified spheroids: round and hard, movable lumps underneath the skin
- Velvety skin
- Hypotonia (poor muscle tone)
- Flat feet
- Frequent bruising
- Displaced (prolapsed) organs
- Hernias

Post-surgery complications can also occur, such as abnormal healing or the protrusion of organs through the surgical site, a condition called postsurgical or incisional hernias.

This subtype can also include heart problems, including:
- Mitral valve prolapse
- Mitral insufficiency
- Aortic dilation.

Mitral valve prolapse (MVP)

Mitral valve prolapse is a "floppy" mitral valve that doesn't close properly. MVP is a very common heart abnormality; according to the National Institutes of Health, about 3% of people in the general population have it. It may not cause symptoms, but if the MVP is causing blood to flow back into the left atrium, it may cause palpitations, irregular heartbeats (arrhythmias) and shortness of breath. The extent of the MVP is measured by how displaced the leaflets (the flaps) are. A displacement of over 2mm is normally cause for concern, as this may lead to increased leaflet thickness, valve-related complications, or mitral insufficiency (Weyman).

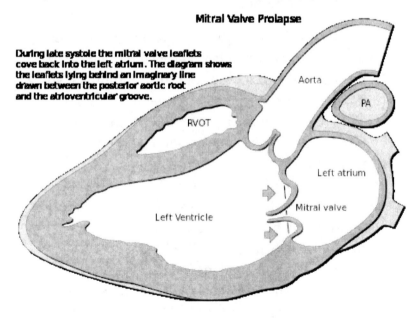

Mitral Valve Prolapse

During late systole the mitral valve leaflets cove back into the left atrium. The diagram shows the leaflets lying behind an imaginary line drawn between the posterior aortic root and the atrioventricular groove.

Aorta

PA

RVOT

Left atrium

Mitral valve

Left Ventricle

Mitral insufficiency

Mitral insufficiency (also called mitral valve regurgitation) is a disorder where the mitral valve does not close properly. The mitral valve separates the upper and lower chambers of the left side of the heart. This can lead to congestive heart failure or severe arrhythmias (problems with your heart's rhythm). Treatment depends on how severe your signs and symptoms are. If you have mild mitral insufficiency, no treatment may be necessary. However, heart surgery to repair the valve may be needed if your signs and symptoms are severe.

Aortic dilation

Aortic dilation is where the aorta becomes enlarged. An aorta that is severely enlarged carries a higher risk for rupturing or tearing. For adults, you'll often hear the aorta measured in millimeters (mm). Anything over 40mm starts to be cause for concern. In children, a *z-score* is usually used to take into account age, height and weight. Z-scores are used in statistics to measure how far from the mean (the average) a certain score is. In pediatric cardiology, z-scores can tell a physician how far a patient's aorta size is from what would be expected in the "average" person of that age, height and weight (Chubb). Z-scores are used because the size of the aorta changes with age and what's more important is the size of the aorta relative to the size of the patient. There are many z-score calculators online that you can use for calculating a pediatric z-score (search for "z score aortic root"). This condition can be treated with surgery.

Hypermobility Type

The hypermobility type of EDS was known as EDS III in the older classification system. The primary symptom is joints that over-extend. Other symptoms that are relatively common with this type are:
- Chronic joint pain
- Easy bruising
- Joint dislocation (especially the jaw, knees and shoulders)
- Skin abnormalities
- Unusually elastic skin
- Velvety skin.

Vascular Type

The vascular type was formerly classified as EDS IV. The main signs and symptoms of this type are:
- Abnormal channels between arteries
- Characteristic facial features such as a thin nose, prominent eyes and hollow cheeks
- Clubfoot
- Early onset varicose veins

- Extremely fragile tissues (including arteries in the bowels) that can rupture easily
- Frequent, severe bruising even from minor accidents or bumps
- Hypermobile joints, especially on the fingers and toes
- Skin that appears prematurely aged
- Unusually low levels of fatty tissue under the skin on the arms, face, feet, hands and legs
- Very thin, transparent skin. The veins under the skin are pronounced, especially over the chest and abdomen.
- Weakening of arterial walls, which can lead to aneurysms.

People with EDS vascular type should be extremely cautious about severe pain in the abdomen or the sides of the body between the ribs and hips. This may indicate arterial or intestinal rupture, which can be a life-threatening emergency.

Pneumohemothorax

People with EDS vascular type are at a higher risk of developing a collapsed lung (pneumothorax).
    A pneumothorax is an abnormal collection of gas or air in the space between the lung and the chest wall that collapses the lung. The pain may resemble a heart attack and can be a medical emergency; if you

suspect you have a pneumothorax, seek immediate medical attention.

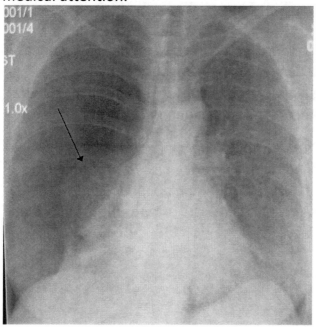

Aneurysms

If you have EDS vascular type, you are at a higher risk for an aneurysm. Although aneurysms are more common in the head and neck, they can occur in other areas.

An aneurysm (AN-u-rism) is a balloon-like bulge in an artery. The arteries are oxygen-rich blood vessels, carrying oxygen to different parts of your body. Arteries have thick walls to resist typical blood pressure level. These arteries may be weaker in vascular type EDS patients. The force of blood pushing against the weakened or injured walls can result in an aneurysm.

An aneurysm is a serious medical problem as it can cause dangerous bleeding inside the body, including a dissection or rupture. If you suspect you have an aneurysm, seek emergency care.

Figure A shows a normal aorta. Figure B shows a thoracic aortic aneurysm (which is located behind the heart). Figure C shows an abdominal aortic aneurysm located below the arteries that supply blood to the kidneys.

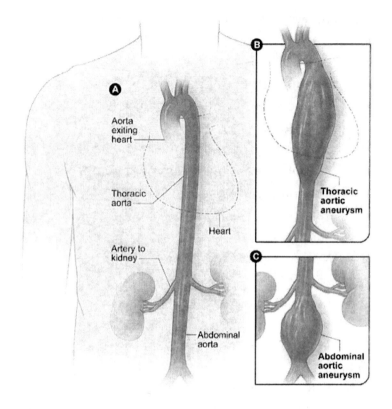

Thoracic aortic aneurysm (TAA)

An aneurysm that occurs in the chest part of the aorta is known as a thoracic aortic aneurysm. Aortic aneurysms can lead to aortic dissection (a tear in the inner wall of the aorta). TAAs are typically are repaired with surgery. Early detection and intervention are critical because aneurysms and dissections can lead to a rupture and massive internal bleeding. Symptoms of an aortic aneurysm can include:

- Pain in your chest, back or neck
- Severe chest/back pain that feels like ripping or tearing. The pain may move around
- Swelling in your head, neck and arms
- Trouble breathing, coughing or wheezing
- Coughing up blood
- Pale skin
- Faint pulse
- Numbness and tingling
- Paralysis
- A fear of impending death.

About 20 percent of people with thoracic aortic aneurysm have a familial history, called familial thoracic aortic aneurysm and dissection (FTAAD). In other words, it runs in the family. The condition does not always cause symptoms, which is why preventative screening is a must.

Abdominal aortic aneurysms (AAAs)

Most abdominal aortic aneurysms (AAAs) happen slowly but surely. They generally do not trigger signs or signs until they rupture. If you have an AAA, your physician could feel a throbbing mass when checking your abdomen.

When signs or symptoms are present, you could have:
- A throbbing sensation in the abdomen.
- Deep pain in your back or your abdomen.
- Steady, gnawing pain within your abdomen that lasts for hours or days.

If an AAA ruptures, signs or symptoms might include:
- Sudden, severe pain inside your abdomen and back.
- Nausea (feeling ill in your stomach) and vomiting.
- Constipation and difficulties with urination.
- Clammy, sweaty skin.
- Light-headedness; along with a rapid heart rate when standing up.

Internal bleeding from a ruptured aorta can send you into shock. If you suspect you have an aneurysm or dissection, this can be life-threatening and requires prompt treatment.

Surgery, such as a Bentall procedure or valve-sparing surgery, is most effective *before* a dissection has happened. A Bentall procedure involves composite graft replacement of the aortic valve, aortic root and ascending aorta, with re-implantation of the coronary arteries into the graft.

Brain Aneurysms

A brain aneurysm is an abnormal bulge or "ballooning" in the wall of an artery in the brain. They are sometimes called berry aneurysms because they are often the size of a small berry. Most brain aneurysms produce no symptoms until they become large, begin to leak blood, or burst.

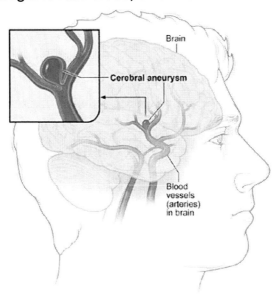

If a brain aneurysm presses on nerves in your brain, it can cause signs and symptoms. These can include:

- A droopy eyelid.
- Double vision or other changes in vision.
- Pain above or behind the eye.
- A dilated pupil.
- Numbness or weakness on one side of the face or body.

Treatment depends on the size and location of the aneurysm, whether it is infected, and whether it has burst. If a brain aneurysm bursts, symptoms can include a sudden, severe headache, nausea and vomiting, stiff neck, loss of consciousness, and signs of a stroke. Any of these symptoms requires immediate medical attention.

Surgery and childbirth with vascular type EDS

People with EDS vascular type are sometimes prone to experiencing complications from surgery, like a condition called dehiscence, which is where the surgical wound separates. Women with EDS vascular type are at a higher risk for certain pregnancy complications, including vaginal tearing and uterine rupture.

Kyphoscoliosis Type

This type (formerly called EDS VI), sometimes has signs and symptoms that are present at birth, including:
- Joints that over-extend
- Poor muscle tone
- Scoliosis (curvature of the spine).

Poor muscle tone (hypotonia) can lead to the delay of developmental milestones involving motor skills and it's common for individuals to lose their ability to walk by the age of 30.

Other signs and symptoms of kyphoscoliosis include:
- A risk of ruptured arteries
- Easy bruising
- Fragile tissues
- Reduced bone mass
- Retinal detachment.

Arthrochalasia Type

This type (formerly called EDS VIIA and VIIB]) normally has the following signs and symptoms:
- Abnormal curvature of the spine from side to side
- Hip dislocation at birth
- Hypermobile joints
- Partial joint dislocation, especially the elbows, feet, knees and hips
- Poor muscle tone
- Reduced bone mass.

Less frequent signs and symptoms include:
- Easily scarred skin
- Easy bruising
- Fragile skin
- Very elastic skin.

Dermatosparaxis Type

Signs and symptoms for dermatosparaxis type (formerly EDS VIIC) include:
- Extensive bruising
- Sagging and soft skin
- Severely fragile skin.

People with this type are sometimes susceptible to hernias.

Other, rarer, forms of EDS are:

EDS periodontosis type (EDS Type VIII) which has signs and symptoms similar to the classical type. In addition people with this type may suffer from premature tooth loss due to the disease affecting the gum tissue.

EDS progeroid form, which is commonly characterized by:
- Degenerative skin scars
- Loose, elastic skin
- Reduced bone mass
- Slow wound healing

People with this type may occasionally have:
- Delayed mental development
- Premature wrinkling of facial skin
- Short stature
- Thin hair on the scalp, eyebrows, and eyelashes.

EDS, cardiac valvular form's common signs and symptoms include:
- Cardiac valve defects
- Elastic skin
- Joints that extend too far.

EDS type IX is now known as *occipital horn syndrome* and EDS type XI is known as *familial hypermobility syndrome.*

CAUSES

Ehlers-Danlos syndrome is a hereditary disorder usually transmitted as an autosomal dominant or autosomal recessive trait.

Autosomal dominant means that you only have to get the gene from one parent to be affected with the disease. Each patient usually only has one parent who is affected, although it is possible for both parents to have EDS.

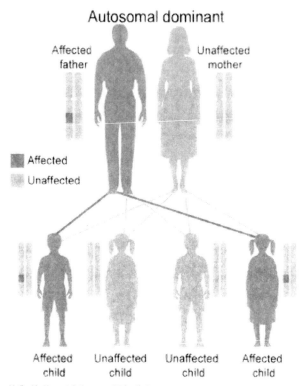

Autosomal dominant

Affected father — Unaffected mother

Affected
Unaffected

Affected child | Unaffected child | Unaffected child | Affected child

U.S. National Library of Medicine

If a person with a dominant gene chooses to have children, they have a 50 percent chance (1 in 2) of having a child with EDS. If you have one child with EDS, that fact does not affect whether a second child has EDS; each child has a 50% chance of acquiring the condition.

With **autosomal recessive**, both genes are faulty. In other words, you inherited a faulty gene from each of your parents. It's possible to carry one copy of the faulty gene, but if the disease follows an autosomal pattern of inheritance then you will be a carrier and will not show signs of the disease. If both parents are carriers, there is a 2 percent chance that any child will carry the disease.

Our bodies contain about 20,000 genes, which are carried on 46 structures called chromosomes. Most chromosome come on pairs (one from each parent), except for the two sex chromosomes, XX for a girl and XY for a boy. The remaining 44 chromosomes which are paired and numbered 1 through 22. Each chromosome has a small arm (P for the French "Petit) and a long Q arm.

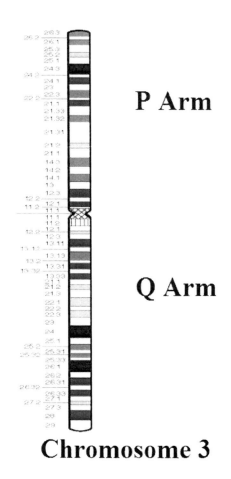

P Arm

Q Arm

Chromosome 3

A common chromosomal disorder is a deletion, where part of the chromosome is missing (deleted).

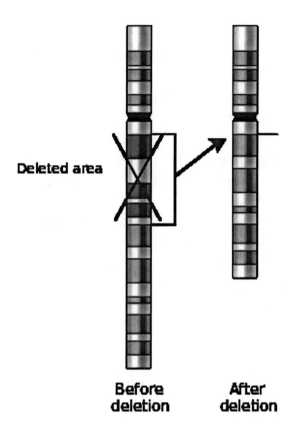

Deleted area

Before
deletion

After
deletion

Geneticists use genetic maps to describe where genes are found on a chromosome. One type of map is called a cytogenetic location, which refers to where a particular band of a lab-stained chromosome lies. For example, the location 3p25-26 refers to Chromosome 3, locations 25-26 on the long (q) arm. A deletion of 3p25 means that part of the gene normally found at 2p25 is missing.

EDS classical type has an autosomal dominant pattern of inheritance.
Around half of all EDS classical types are caused by a defect in one of two genes:
Collagen type V, alpha-1 (COL5A1), found on chromosome 9 (9q34.2-q34.3), and collagen type V, alpha-2 (COL5A2), found on chromosome 2 (2q31).

EDS hypermobility type has an autosomal dominant pattern of inheritance. The specific genes affected are not known although a small number of people have a deficiency of a protein called tenascin X, which is used in building collagen.

EDS vascular type has an autosomal dominant inheritance pattern. This subtype is caused by mutations of collagen type III, alpha-1 (COL3A1), found on the long arm of chromosome 2 (2q31).

EDS kyphoscoliosis type has an autosomal recessive inheritance pattern.
This type is caused by mutations in the PLOD (procollagen-lysine, 2-oxoglutarate 5-dioxygenase) gene that. The PLOD gene has the cytogenetic location (1p36.3-p36.2).

EDS, arthrochalasia type has an autosomal dominant inheritance pattern. This type is caused by mutations in the collagen type I, alpha-1 (COL1A1) gene; this gene is found at cytogenetic location (17q21.31-q22.05). A second gene, collagen type I, alpha-2 (COL1A2) has also been linked to this type. COL1A2 is found on the long arm of chromosome 7 (7q22.1).

EDS dermatosparaxis type has an autosomal recessive pattern of inheritance. This type is thought to be due to mutations genes that encode procollagen I N-terminal peptidase, which modifies collagen.

EDS periodontosis type has an autosomal dominant inheritance pattern.

EDS progeroid type has an autosomal recessive pattern of inheritance; it is caused by mutations in the B4GALT7 gene.

EDS, cardiac valvular type has an autosomal recessive pattern of inheritance. This type is thought to be caused by mutations in the COL1A2 gene.

EDS dysfibronectinemic type, is thought to have an autosomal recessive pattern of inheritance.

EDS type V is an X-linked genetic disorders and occurs mostly in males. As males only have one copy of the X chromosome, a faulty gene means they will develop the disorder.

Females can carry the faulty gene, but usually do not develop the disease.

Diagnosis

When diagnosing EDS, your doctor will perform a physical to look for characteristic signs of EDS. For example, they may want to assess your skin and joints for signs of elastic skin or loose joints. They will also take your personal and family history. They may also order some specialized tests. Which tests are ordered depends on which subtype of EDS your physician thinks you may have. Genetic testing may be a possibility if a specific gene has been identified in your family (this includes prenatal testing and postnatal testing).

A skin biopsy may be ordered for some EDS subtypes in order to look for characteristic abnormalities in collagen structure.

In addition, your doctor may order a CT scan, MRI, or echocardiography to detect mitral valve prolapse or aortic dilatation.

MRI

An MRI is a safe, painless technique to produce detailed 3-D images of your body. Although the test is painless, many people feel claustrophobic during the test, as you'll lay on a stretcher in a tube for the procedure. The machine itself is extremely noisy (you'll hear loud, random banging sounds) and takes around 45 minutes to complete – during which time you'll have to lay completely still. You'll be given ear protection and a "panic button" so that you can alert the technician if you have difficulties during the test. If you have an issue with claustrophobia, you can ask your doctor to provide a mild sedative (like Valium) for the procedure.

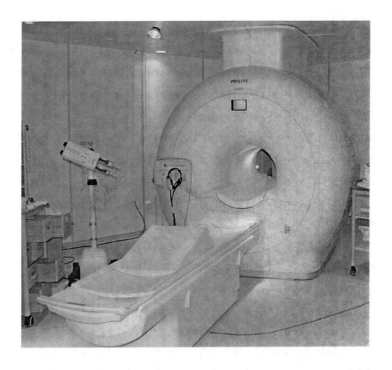

MRIs are extremely safe, and there are no known side effects from the imaging procedure itself. On the rare occasion the machine does cause harm, it's usually unrelated to the imaging itself. Make sure you tell the technician if you have any metal in your body. You'll be given a comprehensive questionnaire when you arrive for the test which will ask about potential objects that can cause issues – make sure you read it completely. Aneurysm clips and pacemakers are just two devices that could cause serious issues. In addition, some MRI accidents have happened because of:

1. Projectiles. The MRI is a giant magnet and on rare occasions, objects have been sucked into the magnetic field..

2. Burns. Don't touch the walls of the MRI tunnel as it carries the risk of severe burns. If there is a risk of you coming into contact with the wall, the technician should place some kind of padding between you and the wall. Despite precautions, there have been some cases of burns being so severe that patients have needed skin grafts.

3. Hearing loss. The machines are very, very loud. You'll be given hearing protection, so make sure you keep it on at all times when in the room.

"It was really tight in the tunnel. So tight that there was only above six inches above my head. But it wasn't as bad as I thought it would be. Both ends were open, so it wasn't quite as claustrophobic as I thought. I was surprised that the table moved – that was a little disconcerting, but the big thing for me is that I had my husband in the room. That made me a bit calmer during the procedure (he could rescue me if I needed!)." Jill—Houston, TX.

CT scan

A CT (computed tomography) scan uses x-rays to create a cross-sectional picture of your body. The test is performed with you lying on a table. You'll be inside the CT scanner, which resembles a large donut. A computer takes the images from the scanner and those images can be viewed on a monitor, stored or printed. The scan usually takes less than 30 minutes.

A CT scan may be used with a contrast dye. This non-toxic dye can be administered orally or intravenously and it will pass out through your stools after the test.

If you are unable to tolerate the contrast dye (for example, if you are allergic to it), your physician may order an MRI instead.

Echocardiogram

An echocardiogram is a sonogram of the heart. This means that it depicts, through images, how the heart is performing. A wand is pressed against the heart and the sound of heartbeat is transmitted through the wand so that they are converted into images. These images show the performance of the heart valves. Through this test, the doctor knows whether the pectus excavatum has caused your heart to beat irregularly or abnormally.

In this test, a dozen leads are attached to the body with the help of a sticky adhesive. This test is helpful in determining that whether the heartbeat is regular or irregular. It also tells that whether the electrical signals which control our heartbeat are functioning normally. The test is painless and takes only a few minutes.

X-Rays
Specialized x-ray studies to detect calcified spheroids or determine the extent of scoliosis and/or kyphosis. X-rays may also be used to check for other abnormalities.

If you have EDS vascular type, your physician may recommend monitoring of your arteries with periodic MRI or other non-invasive imaging. **Angiography**, an invasive procedure, should not be used as it poses significant risks for people with EDS, such as arterial tearing.

Living with EDS

Treatment depends on which type of EDS you have, what symptoms you have and how severe those symptoms are. You may encounter a wide variety of specialists including:

- Pediatricians
- Surgeons
- Physical therapists
- Occupational therapists
- Orthopedists (specialists in disorders of the joints, muscles, skeleton and related tissues
- Dermatologists (skin specialists)
- Rheumatologists (specialists in connective tissue disorders)

- Braces are sometimes use for EDS patients and may be included as part of a physical therapy program to help strengthen muscles and stabilize joints.
  Individuals should avoid contact sports and

sports that may increase the risk of falls, like gymnastics.
- Protective gear, such as shin guards and elbow pads, may benefit some individuals.
- Elective surgery should be avoided because of the risk of wound tearing due to fragile tissues.
- Genetic counseling may benefit affected individuals and family members.

Specific treatments/conditions

Aortic root dilation or aortic dissection

Aortic root surgery may be considered when the diameter of your aortic root is over 5 cm or if you have aortic dissection. Several procedures may be performed, depending on what types of health issues you have and which procedures your surgical team is familiar with. For example, the Button Bentall (simultaneous replacement of the aortic valve, root and the entire ascending aorta) or David valve-sparing procedure (replacement of the aortic root and ascending aorta only) address the aortic valve and root. Button Bentall involves the insertion of a Dacron graft. A David Valve-Sparing procedure can be used if the dilation isn't too extreme; a Dacron graft is still implanted, but the aortic valve is not replaced – it is re-implanted inside the Dacron graft.

You can see a video of a David Procedure here:

http://www.valleyheartandvascular.com/Thoracic-Aneurysm-Program/Video-of-David-Procedure.aspx

In some cases, the decision about which technique to use is sometimes made during the actual surgery. Other, less-common techniques that may be used include:

Yacoub remodeling – a procedure which creates a new aortic root out of Dracon.

Homograft technique – involves replacement of parts with tissue from a cadaver. They are generally used in older patients who have a life-expectancy of less than 15 years.

Prophylactic (preventative) surgery of the aortic root is recommended if:

1. You have a family history of aortic dissection.

2. If the aortic root grows more than 10mm per year.

3. A specific part of your heart (the aortic sinus) is dilated and it involves the ascending aorta.

4. If you have moderate aortic regurgitation or severe mitral regurgitation.

5. If you need major surgery for a non heart-related condition.

6.   If you are thinking about becoming pregnant.

Several other factors may be taken into consideration for prophylactic surgery. The surgery is usually not performed until at least adolescence. It can substantially prolong your life.

Anticoagulant medications such as warfarin are taken for life after artificial heart-valve placement. Warfarin is a medication that helps to prevent blood clots.

What is a Dracon Graft?
A Dacron graft is a man-made (synthetic) material that is used to replace normal body tissues. It is usually made in a tube form to replace or repair blood vessels.

The graft causes very few reactions. It is chemically harmless and easily tolerated by the body. When used in blood vessels, the body eventually grows a new lining to the graft that mimics normal blood vessel linings.

It isn't possible to discuss major heart surgery within the scope of this book. If you are considering heart, surgery, there are many good books available on the subject. We recommend The Open Heart

Companion: Preparation and Guidance for Open-Heart Surgery by Maggie Lichtenberg and Kathleen Blake.

Medications

Beta blockers

Beta blockers help to lower your blood pressure and reduce pressure on your heart. This can help slow down or even prevent aortic dilation and reduce the risk of aortic dissection. Beta-blockers are recommended for older children and adults who have EDS and an enlarged aorta. The optimal age for beta blockers hasn't been established. Some physicians will start beta blockers in infancy; others will monitor your condition until they think beta blockers are necessary. Beta-blockers slow your heart rate and put less stress on the aorta (Shores). Beta-blockers can be considered at any age if you have a dilated aorta. However, the treatment tends to be more effective if the diameter of your aorta is less than 4 cm. ACE inhibitors reduce pressure in your arteries and are sometimes recommended to be used alongside beta blockers.

Angiotensin receptor blockers (ARBs)

One particular ARB, called losartan (Cozaar®), shows promise for preventing aortic growth. At the time of writing, research is being conducted to compare the drug to beta blockers for Marfan syndrome patients (a related disorder) who cannot tolerate beta blockers.

Lens dislocation

Glasses or contact lenses can help restore vision in most cases. Fitting patients with the correct lenses is a challenge with EDS because the optician will need to decide if the glasses should work with your dislocated lens or ignore it. This can be a lengthy procedure involving trial and error. Eyedrops that dilate your pupils may also be prescribed for daily use. Surgery to implant an artificial lens is an option although most experts recommend the surgery is delayed until the eye has stopped growing in the late teens. Replacing the lens is also used for some cases of **cataracts** and other lens-related vision problems.

When is it the right time for surgery?

Whether and when to have surgery is a personal decision. It will very much depend on how much someone's vision loss is affecting their independence and everyday activities. The following factors might play an important role: How good does my eyesight have to be for me to be able to do my job? Are there certain things that I can no longer do, such as reading and sports? Do I have problems finding my way around? Is it becoming too dangerous for me to drive a car?

There is generally no reason to have surgery if a doctor has noticed that the lens is becoming cloudy but it is not yet causing any problems.

In most cases, the timing of surgery will not affect how successful the outcome is: the extent to which the cataract has progressed does not usually influence how well you can see with the newly implanted lens after surgery. But surgery is more difficult if the cataract is very advanced. Eye tests are also no longer as accurate. So it is a good idea to have regular eye tests carried out by an eye doctor (an ophthalmologist). You can then talk to him or her about the right time for surgery.

47

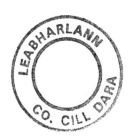

Surgery is only performed on one eye at a time. If both eyes are affected by cataracts or a dislocated lens, one eye is operated after the other.

What should I consider before having surgery?

Another factor that is important for the decision is whether or not someone has other (eye) conditions that could influence the outcome of surgery. Some people also have glaucoma, age-related macular degeneration or eye damage from diabetes. If that is the case, surgery might not clearly improve their vision.

Although most operations do not lead to complications, problems can arise. The eye doctor should thoroughly inform you about the possible advantages and disadvantages of surgery before it is carried out.

What does the surgery involve?

Surgery involves removing the lens and replacing it with an artificial lens. At the beginning of the operation, a small cut is made at the edge of the cornea (the clear covering of the eye). Next, the membrane enclosing the lens is opened at the front. The inner core and outer cortex of the lens are then broken up into small pieces using ultrasound and sucked out through a small cut (phacoemulsification). Once the old lens has been removed in this way, an artificial lens is implanted. The artificial lens lasts a lifetime. Stitches are usually not needed at the end of the operation because the cuts are so small that they normally heal quickly on their own.

The operation takes about 20 to 30 minutes. In most cases it is an outpatient procedure: you can be picked up to go home a few hours after the surgery.

People might stay in the hospital following surgery if they need more intensive care because of other conditions. Talk with your doctor about your EDS to find out if you might have to stay in the hospital after the procedure for monitoring.

What is the most appropriate type of anesthesia?

The surgery can usually be done under local anesthetic. The anesthetic is either given as an injection next to the eye or in the form of eye drops. Both have pros and cons: studies have shown that people who have an injection generally feel less pain during and after surgery. But injections increase the risk of complications.

Pain was experienced during or after surgery by

- 360 out of 1,000 people who had eye drops and

- 130 out of 1,000 people who had an injection.

Anesthesia-related complications:

- About 80 out of 1,000 people who have an injection for cataract surgery are affected by swelling of the conjunctiva, bruising or bleeding in the eye.

- This kind of complication is much less common when eye drops are used, affecting about 1 out of 1,000 people.

The type of anesthetic used probably does not influence how good people's eyesight is after surgery.

Anesthetic eye drops do not affect the eye muscles, so it is possible to move your eyes during surgery. People are therefore asked to look in one direction and keep their eyes still throughout the procedure. Because they need to be very calm and concentrated to do this, anesthetic eye drops are not the right option for everyone, and are only considered for short operations.

How effective is surgery?

About 9 out of 10 people can see better after surgery: they see more clearly and more contrast and are able to see better in dim light too. So surgery can improve your quality of life and make everyday activities easier. Many people are able to do things that were no longer possible, or were difficult, before they had surgery – like driving a car, reading and working at a computer screen. But it can take a few weeks or months for your eyesight to improve as much as possible.

Artificial lenses usually last a lifetime and cannot wear out or become cloudy, so they generally do not have to be replaced. But sometimes a secondary cataract (also known as posterior capsule opacity) develops. This is where people's eyesight gets worse again months or years after surgery because the back of the lens capsule becomes cloudy. It is estimated that about 50 to 100 out of 1,000 people develop secondary cataracts within five years of initial cataract surgery. Secondary cataracts can be treated with a laser.

What are the possible complications?

This type of surgery does not usually cause complications. But inflammations, injuries, bleeding and wound-healing problems are possible. This can lead to vision problems that need to be treated. The most common problems are listed below.

During surgery:

- Damage to the lens capsule: in about 20 to 30 out of 1,000 cases

- Damage to the iris or eyeball: in about 1 to 5 out of 1,000 cases

After surgery:

- Swelling of the retina: in about 20 to 30 out of 1,000 cases

- Lens dislocation: in about 2 to 10 out of 1,000 cases

- Detachment of the retina: in about 2 to 10 out of 1,000 cases

- Inflammation inside of the eye (endophthalmitis): in about 1 to 2 out of 1,000 cases

Some complications are more likely if the eye is anesthetized using an injection. People who have other eye conditions have a higher risk of complications too.

Most complications do not have any long-term consequences. But they can lead to temporary problems such as impaired vision or slower wound healing. People might have to take medication for a while, or further eye surgery might be needed.

The most serious complication is an inflammation inside of the eye. This happens when germs get into the inside of the eye, causing an infection. Symptoms include pain, swelling, a red eye and severe vision problems. If these symptoms arise in the days or weeks following surgery, it is important to see an eye doctor as soon as possible. In the worst case, this kind of inflammation can lead to blindness or loss of the eye, so quick treatment with antibiotics is needed. Bleeding in the eye can cause serious complications too. But bleeding is less common than inflammations inside of the eye, affecting fewer than 1 out of 1,000 people.

How do the artificial lenses differ?

Artificial lenses are also known as intraocular lenses (IOLs). The following different types of lenses are available:

- **Monofocal lenses:** This type of lens allows clear vision at one distance. People have to decide beforehand what kind of monofocal lens they would like, depending on whether they would prefer to have clear vision when looking at things that are far away, at an intermediate distance, or nearby. They can wear glasses to help them see things at other distances. For instance, if someone chooses a lens that allows them to see things that are far away clearly, they will need glasses to read a book.

- **Multifocal lenses:** These lenses allow clear vision both when looking at things that are far away and things that are nearby. People who have multifocal lenses sometimes do not need to wear glasses at all. But their vision might still be blurred when looking at objects at certain distances, and they see somewhat less contrast than people who wear monofocal lenses. Glare is more of a problem with multifocal lenses too, for example when driving at night.

- **Toric lenses:** This type of lens is especially suitable for people who have astigmatism.

Multifocal lenses and toric lenses are more expensive than monofocal lenses. If patients would like to have multifocal or toric lenses, they may have to pay the difference themselves. Because using these types of lenses can be expensive, it is worth carefully weighing the pros and cons of the different types of lenses before making a decision. It might be helpful to get a second opinion from a different eye doctor.

One thing that is more important than the type of lens is the strength (the refractive power) of the lens. The lens must have the right strength for your eye. The eye doctor will do the necessary tests before the operation.

What happens after surgery?

An eye patch should be worn for one day following surgery. The eye might itch, hurt a little, and it might feel like you have something in your eye. These things usually go away again after a few days. Because the eye was recently operated on, it is important not to push on it or rub it, but it is okay to touch it gently. You can return to most everyday activities as usual after a few days, apart from driving a car. It is best to talk to your eye doctor about whether or not to avoid certain activities at first. The doctor will also let you know when your eyesight is good enough for you to start driving again. This is usually possible after a few weeks.

Eye drops are prescribed to be used for some time following surgery, and further follow-up care appointments with your eye doctor are made. Glasses can only be adjusted several weeks after surgery.

If you are thinking about eye surgery...

Make sure your eye surgeon has experience with EDS patients, as you stand a risk of more complications from lens replacement surgery. There are two types of lens replacement (posterior or anterior) and each has their pros and cons. For example, it is easier to surgically implant a lens in the anterior chamber but the lenses may be too small for EDS patientss. Posterior chamber is more difficult but may allow for a better fit. Additionally, there is a higher risk of retinal detachment during posterior chamber surgery. Which technique your eye doctor chooses is usually a matter of their personal choice. Ask your doctor about their reasons for using which type of surgery.

Flat feet (pes planus)

If you have flat feet, you may be able to treat the condition by wearing shoes that have adequate arch support. Sometimes, your doctor may recommend custom orthotics (shoe inserts which are molded to the shape of your feet). Arch supports or custom orthotics don't cure flat feet, but they may help with symptoms which can include knee pain.

Scoliosis

A brace, usually worn for 23 hours a day, is removed only for bathing, showering or swimming. The brace can prevent mild from moderate scoliosis from getting worse, but it cannot treat existing scoliosis or return the spine to "normal." It's worn until growth has stopped, about 14 or 15 for girls and 16 or 17 for boys. How successful the brace is depends on how sever the scoliosis is. For curves over 25 degrees, surgery is usually needed at some point.

In fact, a brace is ineffective for treating severe scoliosis.

You may require surgery for your scoliosis if you are experiencing pain, neurological symptoms or if the curve is extreme (extreme curves over 40 degrees can cause restrictive lung disease). Scoliosis surgery usually isn't performed in children younger than 4 because of the high risk of heart complications. The surgery is performed by straightening the spine and placing metal rods underneath the back muscles. Complications, like the spine not fusing or nerve damage, are rare.

Pneumothorax (collapsed lung)

The treatment of pneumothorax may vary from close observation with early follow-up to immediate needle decompression or insertion of a **chest tube**. Placement of a chest tube is rarely needed and can restore function to your lung. The tube remains in place until your lung heals. However, there is a high risk of recurrence in EDS patients so surgery is usually recommended. The surgery is called thoracoscopy, bleb resection, and talc pleurodesis. With thoracoscopy, a small camera called an endoscope is put into the chest and the bleb (a blister-like pocket of air) is introduced into the chest and the bleb is removed with a surgical tool. A pleurodesis is a procedure that "glues" the lung onto the chest wall.

What does lung surgery involve?

You will receive general anesthesia before surgery. You will be asleep and unable to feel pain. Two common ways to do surgery on your lungs are thoracotomy and video-assisted thoracoscopic surgery (VATS).

Lung surgery using a thoracotomy is called open surgery. In this surgery:

- You will lie on your side on an operating table. Your arm will be placed above your head.
- Your surgeon will make a surgical cut between two ribs. The cut will go from the front of your chest wall to your back, passing just underneath the armpit. These ribs will be separated.
- Your lung on this side will be deflated so that air will not move in and out of it during surgery. This makes it easier for the surgeon to operate on the lung.
- After surgery, one or more drainage tubes will be placed into your chest area to drain out fluids that build up. These tubes are called chest tubes.

- After the surgery on your lungs, your surgeon will close the ribs, muscles, and skin with sutures.
- Open lung surgery may take from 2 to 6 hours.

Video-assisted thoracoscopic surgery:

- Your surgeon will make several small surgical cuts over your chest wall. A videoscope (a tube with a tiny camera on the end) and other small tools will be passed through these cuts.
- One or more tubes will be placed into your chest to drain fluids that build up.
- This procedure leads to much less pain and a faster recovery than open lung surgery.

However, sometimes video surgery may not be possible, and the surgeon may have to switch to an open surgery.

Risks

Risks for any anesthesia include:

- Allergic reactions to medicines
- Breathing problems

Risks for any surgery include:

- Bleeding
- Blood clots in the legs that may travel to the lungs
- Heart attack or stroke during surgery
- Infection, including in the surgical cut, lungs, bladder, or kidney

Risks of this surgery include:

- Failure of the lung to expand
- Injury to the lungs or blood vessels
- Need for a chest tube after surgery
- Pain
- Prolonged air leak
- Repeated fluid buildup in the chest cavity.

Before the Procedure

Smoking isn't recommended if you have EDS. However, if you do smoke, you should stop smoking several weeks before your surgery. Ask your doctor or nurse for help.

Always tell your doctor or nurse:

- What drugs, vitamins, herbs, and other supplements you are taking, even ones you bought without a prescription
- If you have been drinking a lot of alcohol, more than 1 or 2 drinks a day

During the week before your surgery:

- You may be asked to stop taking drugs that make it hard for your blood to clot. Some of these are aspirin, ibuprofen (Advil, Motrin), vitamin E, warfarin (Coumadin), clopidogrel (Plavix), or ticlopidine (Ticlid).
- Ask your doctor which drugs you should still take on the day of your surgery.
- Prepare your home for your return from the hospital.

On the day of your surgery:

- Do not eat or drink anything after midnight the night before your surgery.
- Take the medications your doctor prescribed with small sips of water.
- Your doctor or nurse will tell you when to arrive at the hospital.

After the Procedure

Most people stay in the hospital for 5 to 7 days for open thoracotomy and 1 to 3 days after video-assisted thoracoscopic surgery. You may spend time in the intensive care unit (ICU) after either surgery.

During your hospital stay, you will:

- Be asked to sit on the side of the bed and walk as soon as possible after surgery
- Have tube(s) coming out of the side of your chest to drain fluids
- Wear special stockings on your feet and legs to prevent blood clots
- Receive shots to prevent blood clots
- Receive pain medicine through an IV (a tube that goes into your veins) or by mouth with pills. You may receive your pain medicine through a special machine that gives you a dose of pain medicine when you push a button. This allows you to control how much pain medicine you get.
- Be asked to do a lot of deep breathing to help prevent pneumonia and infection. Deep breathing exercises also help inflate the lung that was operated on. Your chest tube(s) will remain in place until your lung has fully inflated.

Related disorders

Occipital horn syndrome (OHS) was formerly called EDS type IX. The disorder was recategorized as it is linked with copper metabolism. OHS is characterized by:
- Very loose skin
- Bladder abnormalities
- Horn-like bony protuberances on either side of the skull
- Limited extension of elbows and knees
- Other skeletal abnormalities; excessive hypermobile fingers and toes.

Familial hypermobility syndrome , formerly EDS type XI, does not have the joint hypermobility and skin changes seen in EDS, which led to the separate classification.

Symptoms usually include:

- Excessive extension of joints
- Frequent joint dislocations
- Loose joints.

Marfan syndrome

In 1931 Henricus Jacobus Marie Weve coined the term "Marfan Syndrome" to describe a genetic disorder that affects the body's connective tissue. Marfan syndrome (MFS) can result in a myriad of signs and symptoms ranging from extremely long fingers to abnormalities with internal organs, including the heart.

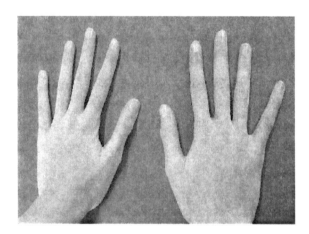

Arachnodactyly

The systems usually affected are the cardiovascular (heart and blood vessels) and ocular (eyes) along with the bones and joints.

Properly treated, and with careful monitoring, people with MFS can have a life-expectancy that's close to a person without MFS. However, it can be a life-threatening condition, even with treatment. For example, if the main blood vessel that carries blood away from the heart (the aorta) is dilated or if there is a bulge in the wall of the aorta (called a *thoracic aortic aneurysm*) this can result in early death.

In Marfan syndrome, there is usually a defect or mutation of the fibrillin-1 (FBN1) gene. The FBN1 gene tells the body how to make the fibrillin-1 protein. The fibrillin-1 protein is responsible for strengthening the body's connective tissue. This mutation causes the body to make too much of another protein called transforming growth factor beta (TGF-β), which results in problems with growth and development.

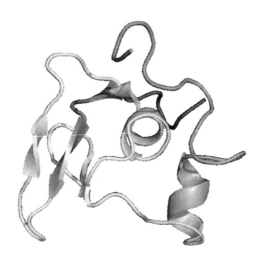

The FBN1 protein

Marfan syndrome is a genetic disease that runs in families. About 75% of people with Marfan syndrome inherit the disorder from their parents. The remaining 25% of patients are thought to have a spontaneous genetic mutation (Loeys et al. 2004, Liu et al. 2001, Turner et al. 2009).

"I was diagnosed with Marfan Syndrome in 2001. Ten years later, a doctor suspected I had a different connective tissue syndrome. A urine test was sent to the lab, and six weeks later I found out I didn't have MFS at all – it turns out I have a rare type of Ehler's Danlos. I'm still stunned that the correct diagnosis wasn't picked up all those years ago." Jill, Cheyenne Wyoming.

Loeys-Dietz Syndrome

Loeys-Dietz Syndrome is another connective-tissue disorder which has many features in common with Marfan syndrome. In fact, it has so many features in common with MFS that it was once called (prior to about 2006) Marfan Syndrome Type II. It is more lethal than MFS and carries a high risk of aortic aneurysms and complications during pregnancy. The genes affected are TGFBR1, TGFBR2 or SMAD3. There are three types of the syndrome.

Loeys-Dietz Syndrome Type I is characterized by an enlarged aorta, which may lead to aortic dissection or aortic aneurysm. Like MFS, Loeys-Dietz Syndrome Type I patients may also have aneurysms or dissections in other parts of the body. Arteries may have abnormal twists and turns, a condition called arterial tortuosity. Other conditions associated with Type I include:

- Widely spaced eyes
- A split in the soft flap of tissue at the back of the mouth
- Cleft palate (an opening in the roof of the mouth)
- A tendency to bruise easily and develop abnormal scars

- Premature fusion of the skull bones
- Scoliosus
- Pectus excavatum or pectus carinatum
- Club feet
- Elongated limbs with joint deformities

Loeys-Dietz Syndrome Type II has many of the features of Type I, such as arterial tortuosity, an enlarged aorta, a tendency to bruise easily and abnormal scarring. Skeletal problems tend not to be so severe. Skin problems characterize this type: skin may be velvety and translucent, so that the underlying veins are visible.

Loeys-Dietz Syndrome Type III is characterized by aortic and arterial aneurysms plus osteoarthritis (pain in the joints). This type is sometimes called aneurysms-osteoarthritis syndrome.

Ectopia Lentis Syndrome

People who inherit the skeletal features of MFS (like a tall thin body type and long arms and fingers) but do not have any other features of MFS such as aortic dilation may be diagnosed with ectopic lentis syndrome (sometimes called familial ectopia lentis) if they have lens dislocation of the eye. The only way a diagnosis can be made between the two syndromes is by frequent monitoring (i.e. echocardiograms) to rule out Marfan syndrome.

Beals Syndrome (Congenital contractural arachnodactyly)

Like EDS, Beals syndrome is an inherited connective tissue disorder with an autosomal dominant pattern of inheritance. For many years, it was thought that Beals syndrome and Marfan syndrome were the same disorder until the discovery that the two disorders were caused by mutations in different genes; Marfan syndrome is caused by a mutation in the FBN1 gene and Beals is caused by mutations in the FBN2 gene. It shares some common characteristics with MFS, including arachnodactyl, kyphoscoliosis, a highly arched palate, myopia and mitral valve prolapse. In very rare cases, people with Beals syndrome may also have aortic dilation. However, there are many features not seen in MFS, including permanently fixed fingers (camptodactyl), "crumpled" ears and permanently fixed joints in a flexed position. Beals syndrome is extremely rare, but how many people are affected is not known.

Familial Thoracic Aortic Aneurysm and Dissection (Familial TAAD)

Familial TAAD is a disorder usually involving the upper part of the aorta (the thoracic aorta). In some cases, the abdominal aorta may be affected or individuals may have brain aneurysms. People with TAAD can have aortic dilation, aneurysms and aortic dissection. However, unlike EDS, no other symptoms are usually involved with familial TAAD. Rarely, people with familial TAAD might have scoliosis, a purplish skin coloration or a pouching in the lower abdomen (inguinal hernia).

Fragile X Syndrome

Fragile X syndrome is a genetic disorder that causes many developmental problems such as cognitive impairment and learning disabilities. Individuals who have fragile X may also have heart problems like aortic root dilation or mitral valve prolapse (Sreeram) and joint laxity (Dietz). However, EDS does typically not cause the types of developmental problems seen in Fragile X.

Gigantism and Acromegaly

Gigantism and acromegaly both cause excessive growth. They are both caused by the production of too much growth hormone. Gigantism causes a high linear growth, resulting in a tall stature while acromegaly causes the bones to increase in size. Acromegaly usually affects middle-aged people while gigantism is seen in childhood and can co-exist with Marfan syndrome. Untreated gigantism and acromegaly can lead to heart problems, including heart failure due to an enlarged heart.

Hyperpituitarism

Hyperpituitarism is an overactive pituitary gland. The pituitary gland plays a role in a wide variety of biological functions, including metabolism, growth, sexual function and blood pressure. Three hormones are oversecreted, including adrenocorticotropic hormone (ACTH). Excess ACTH can result in gigantism.

Hyperthyroidism

Hyperthyroidism is where your thyroid gland produces too much of a hormone called thyroxine. Symptoms include weight loss, sweating, a rapid or irregular heartbeat and nervousness and irritability. It is not a genetic disorder but can be a differential diagnosis for MFS. A differential diagnosis is a diagnostic method to identify the presence of a disease or disorder where several others are possible.

Klinefelter Syndrome

Klinefelter syndrome is a genetic disorder that only affects males. It affects the X chromosome, but it is not inherited. Small testes that don't produce as much testosterone as usual is characteristic of the condition. Like MFS, people with this syndrome tend to be taller than their peers. However, Klinefelter causes a wide range of symptoms that are not associated with MFS, including reproductive issues, breast enlargement and delayed or incomplete puberty.

Bicuspid Aortic Valve

A Bicuspid aortic valve is an aortic valve that has two leaflets instead of the normal three. Like EDS, it can cause an enlarged aorta. However, no other EDS-like symptoms and signs are associated with this disorder. It is the most common congenital heart disease and it often runs in families.

MASS Phenotype

Like EDS, MASS phenotype is a disorder of connective tissues. MASS stands for Mitral valve, Aorta, Skin and Skeletal. People with MASS phenotype may have mitral valve prolapsed, a large aortic root diameter, stretch marks on the skin and Marfan-like skeletal features including scoliosis, pectus excavatum or pectus carinatum. However, people with MASS syndrome do not have lens dislocation in the eye or a progression of aortic root dilation to aneurysms or the potential for aortic root dissection.

Schprintzen-Goldberg Syndrome

People with Schprintzen-Goldberg Syndrome have many Marfan-like features, including arachnodactyly, very long limbs, pectus excavatum, pectus carinatum and scoliosis. However, people Schprintzen-Goldberg Syndrome often have delayed development and mild to moderate intellectual disability. They may also have distinctive facial features including widely spaced eyes, protruding eyes, a small lower jaw and ears that are rotated back and low set. This syndrome is caused by mutations in the SKI gene.

Stickler Syndrome

Stickler syndrome is a group of hereditary conditions characterized by a distinctive, flattened facial appearance, eye abnormalities, hearing loss, and joint problems. Like EDS, Stickler syndrome can cause retinal detachment, loose joints, scoliosis and kyphosis. Other features of Stickler syndrome that are not seen in EDS include hearing loss.

Clinical Trials

Clinical trials are being conducted at the NIH Clinical Center in Bethesda, MD.

Tollfree: (800) 411-1222
TTY: (866) 411-1010
Email: prpl@cc.nih.gov

Clinical trials sponsored by private sources are generally posted at:
www.centerwatch.com

Ehler Danlos Related Organizations

American Heart Association
8200 Brookriver Drive
Suite N-100
Dallas, TX 75247
Phone #: 214-784-7212 or 800-242-8721
Home page: http://www.americanheart.org
Coalition for Heritable Disorders of Connective Tissue (CHDCT)
4301 Connecticut Avenue, NW Suite 404
Washington, DC 20008
Phone #: 202-362-9599 or 800-778-7171
e-mail: chdct@pxe.org
Home page: http://www.chdct.org

Genetic and Rare Diseases (GARD)
Information Center
    PO Box 8126
    Gaithersburg, MD 20898-8126
    Phone #: 301-251-4925 or 888-205-2311
    Home page:
    http://rarediseases.info.nih.gov/GARD/About
    GARD.aspx
National Scoliosis Foundation
    5 Cabot Place
    Stoughton, MA 02072
    Phone #: 781-341-8333 or 800-673-6922
    Home page: http://www.scoliosis.org
NIH/National Institute of Arthritis and
Musculoskeletal and Skin Diseases
    Information Clearinghouse
    One AMS Circle
    Bethesda, MD 20892-3675 USA
    Phone #: 301-495-4484 or 877-226-4267
    Home page: http://www.niams.nih.gov/

REFERENCES

AHA guidelines J Am Dent Assoc, Vol 138, No 6, 739-760.
Wood J et. al. Pulmonary Disease in Patients with Marfan Syndrome. *Thorax* (British Medical Journal). 1984 39:780-784.
Berkow R., ed. The Merck Manual-Home Edition.2nd ed. Whitehouse Station, NJ: Merck Research Laboratories; 2003:1608-9.
Channell K. Marfan syndrome. Emedicine Journal http://www.emedicine.com/orthoped/topic414.htm. Updated April 9, 2010. Accessed June 8, 2011.

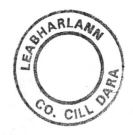

Chen H. Genetics of Marfan Syndrome. Medscape. http://emedicine.medscape.com/article/94631 5-overview

Chen H. Marfan syndrome. Emedicine Journal. http://www.emedicine.com/ped/topic1372.ht m. Updated March 10, 2010. Accessed June 8, 2011.

Chubb, H & Simpson, J. The use of z-scores in pediatric cardiology. Ann Pediatr Cardiol. 2012 Jul-Dec; 5(2): 179–184.

Forteza A, Cortina JM, Sanchez V, et al. Aortic valve preservation in Marfan syndrome. Initial experience. Rev Esp Cardiol. 2007;60:471-5.

GeneTests Website: www.genetests.org

Jones KL. Ed. Smith's Recognizable Patterns of Human Malformation. 5th ed. W. B. Saunders Co., Philadelphia, PA; 1997:546.

Judge DP, Deitz HC. Marfan's syndrome. Lancet. 2005;366:1965-76.
Gott VL, Cameron DE, Alejo DE, et al. Aortic root replacement in 271 Marfan patients: a 24-year experience. Ann Thorac Surg. 2002;73:438-43.

Le Parc JM, Molcard S Tubach F, et al. Marfan syndrome and fibrillin disorders. Joint Bone Surg. 2000;67:401-7.

Le Parc J-M. Marfan syndrome. Orphanet encyclopedia, February 2005. Available at:

http://www.orpha.net/data/patho/GB/Marfan
-interm.htm. Accessed June 8, 2011.

Marfan, Antoine (1896). "Un cas de déformation congénitale des quartre membres, plus prononcée aux extrémitiés, caractérisée par l'allongement des os avec un certain degré d'amincissement" [A case of congenital deformation of the four limbs, more pronounced at the extremities, characterized by elongation of the bones with some degree of thinning].*Bulletins et memoires de la Société medicale des hôspitaux de Paris* **13** (3rd series): 220–226.

National Institutes of Health. What is Mitral Valve Prolapse? www.nhlbi.nih.gov/health/health-topics/topics/mvp/

National Institutes of Health: Aneurysm http://www.nhlbi.nih.gov/health/health-topics/topics/arm/livingwith.html. Accessed August 9, 201.

Neptune, E. What is the appropriate treatment for restrictive lung disease? The Marfan Foundation. https://www.youtube.com/watch?v=0Llw7hfvl tM

Online Mendelian Inheritance in Man (OMIM). The Johns Hopkins University. Loeys-Dietz Syndrome, Type 2B; LDS2B (Marfan Syndrome, Type II, Formerly). Entry No: 610380. Last

Updated July 6, 2010. Available at:
http://www.ncbi.nlm.nih.gov/omim/. Accessed
June 8, 2011.

Ramirez F, Dietz HC. Marfan syndrome: from
molecular pathogenesis to clinical treatment.
Curr Opin Genet Dev. 2007;17:252-8.

Sakai LY, Keene DR, Engvall E. Fibrillin, a new 350-kD
glycoprotein, is a component of extracellular
microfibrils. J Cell Biol. 1986;103:2499-509.

Schievink WI, Parisi JE, Piepgras DG, Michels VV.
Intracranial aneurysms in Marfan's syndrome:
an autopsy study. *Neurosurgery*.. 1997;41:866–
871.

Shores J, Berger KR, Murphy EA and Pyeritz RE.
Progression of aortic dilation and the benefit

Singh KK, Rommel K, Mishra A, Karck M, Haverich A,
Schmidtke J, Arslan-Kirchner M. (2006) TGFβR1
and TGFβR2 mutations in patients with
features of Marfan syndrome and Loeys-Dietz
syndrome. Human Mutation Jun 23

Sports Illustrated. Larger than real life. July 04, 2011.
http://sportsillustrated.cnn.com/vault/article/
magazine/MAG1187806/3/index.htm

Sreeram et. al. Cardiac Abnormalities in the fragile X
Syndrome. Br Heart J 1989; 61-289-91.

Weyman, A & Scherrer-Crosbie, M. Marfan syndrome
and mitral valve prolapse. *J Clin
Invest*. 2004;114(11):1543–1546.

Images
    Aorta: Edorado | Wikimedia Commons
    Aortic valve micrograph: Nephron | Wikimedia
Commons
    FBN1: EMW | Wikimedia Commons
    Slit Lamp: SchuminWeb | Wikimedia Commons
    MVP: Patrick J. Lynch | Wikimedia Commons
    Cataract: EyeMD | Wikimedia Commons

CPSIA information can be obtained at www.ICGtesting.com
Printed in the USA
LVOW10s1023210615

443286LV00019B/1177/P